REMEDIES FOR LIVER CIRRHOSIS

Effective remedies for liver cirrhosis and safety guide on how to go about it.

Dr. John Donald

Table of Contents

CHAPTER ONE

WHAT IS LIVER CIRRHOSIS

Cirrhosis is an overdue degree of scarring (fibrosis) of the liver as a result of many sorts of liver sicknesses and situations, such as hepatitis and persistent alcoholism.

Each time your liver is injured whether by using ailment, excessive alcohol intake or some other purpose it attempts to repair itself. In the procedure, scar tissue forms. As cirrhosis progresses, more and more scar tissue paperwork, making it hard for the liver to feature (decompensate cirrhosis). Advanced cirrhosis is existence-threatening.

The liver damage executed by using cirrhosis normally cannot be undone. But if liver cirrhosis is identified early and the purpose is treated, further damage can be confined and, not often, reversed.

SYMPTOMS OF THE LIVER CIRRHOSIS

Cirrhosis regularly has no signs and symptoms or signs until liver harm is extensive. When symptoms and signs do arise, they will include:

- Fatigue

- Easily bleeding or bruising

- Loss of appetite

- Nausea

- Swelling for your legs, feet or ankles (edema)

- Weight loss

- Itchy pores and skin

- Yellow discoloration within the skin and eyes (jaundice)

- Fluid accumulation for your stomach (ascites)

- Spiderlike blood vessels on your skin

- Redness in the fingers of the palms

- For women, absent or lack of durations now not associated with menopause

- For guys, loss of intercourse power, breast enlargement (gynecomastia) or testicular atrophy

- Confusion, drowsiness and slurred speech (hepatic encephalopathy).

CAUSES

A wide range of diseases and conditions can damage the liver and result in cirrhosis.

Some of the reasons encompass:

- Chronic alcohol abuse

- Chronic viral hepatitis (hepatitis B, C and D)

- Fat accumulating within the liver (nonalcoholic fatty liver disease)

- Iron buildup within the body (hemochromatosis)

- Cystic fibrosis

- Copper accumulated in the liver (Wilson's sickness)

- Poorly fashioned bile ducts (biliary atresia)

- Alpha-1 antitrypsin deficiency

- Inherited disorders of sugar metabolism (galactosemia or glycogen garage ailment)

- Genetic digestive ailment (Alagille syndrome)

• Liver disease resulting from your frame's immune gadget (autoimmune hepatitis)

• Destruction of the bile ducts (primary biliary cirrhosis)

• Hardening and scarring of the bile ducts (primary sclerosing cholangitis

• Infection, together with syphilis or brucellosis

• Medications, including methotrexate or isoniazid

Risk factors

• Drinking an excessive amount of alcohol. Excessive alcohol consumption is a hazard issue for cirrhosis.

• Being obese. Being overweight increases your threat of conditions that could result in cirrhosis, such as nonalcoholic fatty liver sickness and nonalcoholic steatohepatitis.

• Having viral hepatitis. Not every body with chronic hepatitis will broaden cirrhosis, however it is one of the international's leading reasons of liver disorder.

Complications

Complications of cirrhosis can consist of:

• High blood stress in the veins that supply the liver (portal hypertension).Cirrhosis slows the regular flow of blood thru the liver, hence increasing pressure within the vein that brings blood to the liver from the intestines and spleen.

• Swelling in the legs and abdomen. The extended pressure in the portal vein can motive fluid to build up within the legs (edema) and inside the abdomen (ascites). Edema and ascites additionally may also result from the inability of the liver to make enough of sure blood proteins, which include albumin.

• Enlargement of the spleen (splenomegaly). Portal high blood pressure also can cause adjustments to and swelling of the spleen, and trapping of white blood cells and platelets. Decreased white blood cells and platelets for your blood can be the first signal of cirrhosis.

• Bleeding. Portal high blood pressure can reason blood to be redirected to smaller veins. Strained by using the greater stress, those smaller veins can burst, causing extreme bleeding. Portal hypertension might also purpose enlarged veins (varices) in the esophagus (esophageal varices) or the belly (gastric varices) and lead to existence-threatening bleeding. If the liver cannot make enough clotting elements, this also can make contributions to persevered bleeding.

• Infections. If you have cirrhosis, your body may additionally have issue preventing infections. Ascites can lead to bacterial peritonitis, a severe infection.

• Malnutrition. Cirrhosis may also make it more hard for your body to manner vitamins, leading to weakness and weight reduction.

• Buildup of pollutants within the mind (hepatic encephalopathy). A liver damaged by using cirrhosis isn't able to clear pollutants from the blood as well as a healthy liver can. These toxins can then increase within the brain and reason intellectual confusion and problem concentrating. With time, hepatic encephalopathy can development to unresponsiveness or coma.

• Jaundice. Jaundice occurs while the diseased liver doesn't remove sufficient bilirubin, a blood waste product, from your blood. Jaundice reasons yellowing of the pores and skin and whites of the eyes and darkening of urine.

• Bone disease. Some people with cirrhosis lose bone energy and are at more hazard of fractures.

• Increased danger of liver cancer. A huge share of those who develop liver most cancers have pre-existing cirrhosis.

• Acute-on-persistent cirrhosis. Some human beings come to be experiencing multiorgan failure. Researchers now believe this is a distinct difficulty in some humans who've cirrhosis, but they don't absolutely apprehend its causes.

CHAPTER TWO

PREVENTION

Reduce your risk of cirrhosis with the aid of taking those steps to take care of your liver:

•   Do not drink alcohol if you have cirrhosis. If you have liver disease, you have to keep away from alcohol.

•   Eat a healthful weight-reduction plan. Choose a plant-primarily based diet that is complete of end result and greens. Select whole grains and lean sources of protein. Reduce the quantity of fatty and fried ingredients you devour.

•   Maintain a healthy weight. An excess amount of body fats can harm your liver. Talk for your health practitioner about a weight loss plan if you are overweight or overweight.

• Reduce your danger of hepatitis. Sharing needles and having unprotected intercourse can boom your risk of hepatitis B and C. Ask your doctor about hepatitis vaccinations.

If you are involved about your danger of liver cirrhosis, communicate in your doctor approximately methods you could lessen your hazard.

Cirrhosis is the end result of long-term, non-stop damage to the liver and may be because of many one-of-a-kind causes. The harm ends in scarring, known as fibrosis. Irregular bumps (nodules) replace the clean liver tissue and the liver becomes tougher. Together, the scarring and the nodules are referred to as cirrhosis.

Cirrhosis can take a few years to develop and might accomplish that without any substantial symptoms until the harm to the liver may be very critical. The construct-up of scar tissue can intervene with the waft of blood on your liver and stop it from functioning well. Cirrhosis can lead to liver failure.

HOW NOT UNUSUAL IS CIRRHOSIS?

No one knows for sure what numbers of human beings in the UK have cirrhosis as the majority do no longer understand they have got it till the circumstance is critical. However, there's no doubt that the variety of people with the situation maintains to boom.

Every year over four,000 humans inside the UK die from cirrhosis. Around 700 humans need to have a liver transplant every year to continue to exist.

WHO IS VULNERABLE TO CIRRHOSIS?

Cirrhosis can affect each person – women and men, old and young. People most susceptible to cirrhosis:

- drink too much alcohol

- have a protracted-time period liver contamination, inclusive of Hepatitis B or Hepatitis C

- have an inherited liver disease, along with Haemochromatosis

- have an immune system trouble that results in liver ailment

- are clinically overweight or obese and have a fatty liver

CHAPTER THREE

SYMPTOMS

You are not probable to sense any symptoms of cirrhosis early on. In reality, many humans with cirrhosis best find out in the course of checks for an unrelated contamination. Additionally, the signs and symptoms may be very non-precise, which means that they are additionally resulting from other situations not associated with cirrhosis.

If you've got cirrhosis, you could expand one or extra of the symptoms underneath. If you have got or are involved about any of those symptoms speak them with your health practitioner.

EARLY SYMPTOMS

- usually feeling ill and worn-out all of the time

- lack of urge for food

- loss of weight and muscle losing

- feeling unwell (nausea) and vomiting

- tenderness/pain inside the liver region

- spider-like small blood capillaries at the skin above waist degree (spider angiomas)

- blotchy purple palms

- disturbed sleep pattern

Later symptoms, because the liver is suffering to characteristic

- intensely itchy pores and skin

- yellowing of the whites of the eyes and the skin (jaundice)

- white nails

- ends of hands turn out to be wider/thicker (clubbed palms)

- hair loss

- swelling of the legs, ankles, toes (oedema)

- swelling of the abdomen (ascites)

- dark urine

- pale-colored stools or very darkish/black tarry stools

- frequent nosebleeds and bleeding gums

- easy bruising and diffi culty in preventing small bleeds

- vomiting blood

- common muscle cramps

- right shoulder pain

- in men: enlarged breasts and shrunken testes

- in girls: abnormal or lack of menstrual durations

- impotence and loss of sexual desire

- dizziness and severe fatigue (anaemia)

- shortness of breath

- very fast heartbeat (tachycardia)

- fevers with excessive temperature and shivers

- forgetfulness, memory loss, confusion and drowsiness

- subtle change in personality

- trembling palms

- writing will become difficult, spidery and small

- brilliant gait when on foot; tendency to fall

- increased sensitivity to tablets, both scientific and leisure

- extended sensitivity to alcohol

Red flag signs and symptoms

If you have got any of the subsequent signs and symptoms you have to see a doctor straight away, specially when you have lately been identified with cirrhosis:

- fever with excessive temperatures and shivers, regularly because of an infection

- shortness of breath

- vomiting blood

- very darkish or black tarry stools (faeces)

- durations of mental confusion or drowsiness.

Although those signs might also appear very exclusive, because your liver is chargeable for so many one of a kind functions, if it stops running properly, various troubles can end result.

Yellow eyes or pores and skin

If your pores and skin and the whites of your eyes turn yellow you could have jaundice.

Two matters can motive jaundice:

• a blockage (obstruction) in the bile duct

• harm for your liver or some disorder affecting the liver so that it cannot cope with bilirubin, a derivative of the breakdown of vintage pink blood cells.

If either of these occurs, bilirubin – that's yellow – flows back into the blood and indicates up in the skin and the eyes.

Swollen stomach and legs

Swelling in your stomach is referred to as ascites. The swelling is caused by fluid constructing up in the lining around your abdomen. This can take place slowly over weeks or months and may be painful, mainly if the fluid will become infected and requires pressing interest.

You might also get swelling for your legs, ankles or ft, known as peripheral oedema.

Fever with high temperatures and shivers

People with cirrhosis are susceptible to infections, which could make their liver situation worse. As a result, they ought to are seeking clinical interest if they increase a temperature.

Tarry black stools or vomiting blood

Internal bleeding because of liver harm is regularly first observed in very darkish or black tarry faeces (maelena) and the vomiting of blood (haematemesis). Having both of those signs and symptoms will need urgent clinical interest.

If your liver is badly scarred from tremendous fibrosis or cirrhosis, blood will be not able to waft thru it effortlessly. As a end result, stress builds up inside the vein that includes blood to the liver from the gut – the portal vein.

Having excessive blood strain in the portal vein is called portal hypertension. As the pressure mounts, blood starts offevolved to back up. It unearths any other way of reaching the coronary heart via the usage of more veins lining your oesophagus and stomach referred to as varices. Varices have fragile walls, which can't easily manage the increased blood float and often burst, leading to inner bleeding.

This blood loss may additionally simply be a mild ooze, resulting in symptoms of anaemia that encompass tiredness and shortness of breath, but every now and then there may be foremost bleeding, with a haemorrhage and vomiting of blood. Haemorrhaging varices are a extreme and lifestyles-threatening problem of cirrhosis and need emergency scientific treatment.

Memory loss and confusion (Encephalopathy)

Confusion, short-time period reminiscence troubles or even lack of focus can end result if your liver is not working nicely. You might feel sleepy, experience tremors and have issue acting simple duties. This is because the liver, while operating properly, receives rid of waste products. When it is broken, the waste products are carried to the brain by using your blood. This circumstance is called encephalopathy.

DIAGNOSIS

It is not continually clean to diagnose cirrhosis. A health practitioner will take a careful scientific history, perform a physical exam and make plans for in addition tests.

The checks for cirrhosis encompass:

• blood checks, which amongst other matters degree the liver function and damage. These are most commonly Liver Function Tests (LFTs). These are used to benefit an idea of ways the one-of-a-kind components of your liver are functioning.

The liver function check is made of a number of separate examinations, each searching at one of a kind properties of your blood. It is used to advantage an indication of ways much your liver is infected or unable to work properly. The check will measure, as an instance, stages of the liver enzymes ALT and AST as these are multiplied at some stage in inflammation (hepatitis).

It will even examine how well your blood clots (referred to as INR time) and how properly your kidneys dispose of a product called creatinine. These are exact indicators for how nicely your liver is operating, and the way this is affecting the relaxation of your body.

• imaging checks wherein your liver may be scanned using ultrasound, computerised tomography (CT) or magnetic resonance imaging (MRI).

Ultrasound, the same technology used to confirm all is properly in being pregnant, sends sound waves into your frame. The echoes are picked up and used to construct a picture of the situation of the liver.

MRI and CT provide an in depth view of your inner organs and are able to generate very distinct go-sectioned pics (or 'slices') of your body area.

• liver biopsy wherein a tiny piece of the liver is taken to be looked at beneath a microscope. A quality hollow needle is surpassed thru the pores and skin into the liver and a small pattern is withdrawn. The check is generally achieved beneath nearby anaesthetic and may mean an in a single day stay in clinic, although most of the people are allowed domestic later the same day if they live nearby.

• endoscopy wherein, following sedation, a skinny bendy tube with a mild and a tiny digital camera on the give up (endoscope) is surpassed down your oesophagus and into your stomach. This is to test for varices in the oesophagus or belly which might also rupture and unexpectedly bleed.

WHAT ARE THE SPECIAL RANGES OF CIRRHOSIS?

Cirrhosis is every so often known as end degree liver disorder. This sincerely method it comes after the alternative stages of liver harm that may consist of irritation (hepatitis), fatty deposits (steatosis) and accelerated stiffness and mild-scarring of your liver (fibrosis).

Many human beings with cirrhosis can sense pretty well and stay for many years while not having a liver transplant. This is due to the fact the liver can characteristic highly properly even when it's far pretty critically damaged.

Cirrhosis is classified as compensated or decompensated. Compensated cirrhosis is where the liver is managing the harm and retaining its essential capabilities. In decompensated cirrhosis, the liver isn't capable of perform all its capabilities competently. People with decompensated liver ailment or cirrhosis regularly have critical signs and headaches including portal hypertension, bleeding varices, ascites and encephalopathy.

There are also structures for grading cirrhosis in line with its severity. One of these is the Childs Pugh Score, which uses signs inclusive of encephalopathy and ascites collectively with blood take a look at consequences for bilirubin, albumin and clotting, to grade cirrhosis from A (particularly slight) to C (extreme). There are different systems including meld (version of stop-degree liver ailment) which can be used to assist decide which sufferers maximum urgently need liver transplants. It makes use of blood take a look at outcomes for bilirubin, creatinine and clotting (INR).

Anything that ends in the long-term, non-stop damage of the liver can reason cirrhosis. These include:

• alcohol

• viral infections including Hepatitis B and Hepatitis C

• a building up of fats within the liver called Non-Alcohol Related Fatty Liver disorder (NAFLD) that could progress to a extra extreme circumstance called non alcoholic steatohepatitis or NASH

• Autoimmune Hepatitis

• Primary Biliary Cholangitis/Cirrhosis (PBC) and other lengthy-term diseases of the bile ducts consisting of Primary Sclerosing Cholangitis (PSC) or Biliary Atresia (BA) in youngsters

• sure inherited sicknesses, including Haemochromatosis and Wilson's disorder

• lengthy-time period contact with a few drugs and poisons

• blood vessel (vascular) sickness, which includes Budd-Chiari Syndrome.

Treatment

Treatment relies upon on the reason and stage of the cirrhosis. The intention of treatment is to prevent the cirrhosis getting worse, to opposite any damage (if this is viable) and to treat any disabling or

existence-threatening complications.

Stopping the progression

Making lifestyle modifications and reducing alcohol out of your weight loss program may additionally assist put off development.

Many reasons of liver disease can now be handled a great deal more successfully than earlier than to prevent or at least slow down any decline in the situation of your liver.

This consists of treating infections such as hepatitis B or C with new anti-viral medicinal drugs and autoimmune diseases consisting of Autoimmune Hepatitis (AIH) with steroid-primarily based tablets. Genetic

Haemochromatosis (GH), an inherited liver sickness, can be managed effectively with phlebotomy or venesection, a system just like blood donation wherein a quantity of blood is frequently taken from a vein to your arm.

CHAPTER FOUR

REVERSING THE TROUBLE

till lately, it was idea that a liver with cirrhosis couldn't be healed. This is usually the case due to the fact maximum diseases that cause scarring of your liver (fibrosis) are long-time period and hard to 'remedy'.However, current research has shown that it can be viable to heal scarring and even cirrhosis in which the liver sickness causing this damage is able to be efficiently treated.

The treatment of Hepatitis B and C, as already noted, offers hope for the development of latest drugs to combat scarring of the liver. More studies, but, needs to be accomplished earlier than any

new remedies become widely to be had.

Treating and dealing with the results of cirrhosis

Another element of remedy is to cope with the complications of cirrhosis as early as viable. For this reason your doctor can also endorse you've got regular tests to pick out problems even earlier than you be aware any signs and symptoms. You can also be given other drugs to reduce blood pressure, to prevent and treat infections and to assist aid your frame's functions.

Portal high blood pressure and variceal bleeding

Medicines such as beta blockers along with propranolol can reduce the chance of bleeding and reduce the severity of any bleed, ought to it arise. If there is a extreme bleed, preliminary remedy is to update the fluid and then to become aware of and accurate the motive of bleeding.

There are several techniques geared toward stemming the bleeding which contain endoscopy.

One of these is referred to as banding, in which a single vein (referred to as an oesophageal varix) is sucked into a ring at the stop of the endoscope. A small band is then positioned around the base of the varix that allows you to manage the bleeding.

Injection sclerotherapy is also used and involves injecting a substance into the veins of the gullet to induce clotting and scar tissue with the intention to assist prevent the veins from bleeding.

If bleeding can't be stopped with the aid of endoscopy, a Sengstaken tube is handed down the throat into the belly. This tool has balloons which as soon as inflated, positioned pressure on the varices and assist manage the bleeding. People are heavily sedated for this system.

If bleeding nevertheless can not be controlled a manner to lower pressure in the portal vein known as a transjugular intrahepatic portosystemic stent shunt (TIPSS) may be wished. In this technique a metallic tube (stent) is surpassed across your liver to join big veins (the portal vein and hepatic vein). This creates a pass (shunt) so the blood flows immediately into the hepatic vein relieving the strain which reasons the varices.

ASCITES AND PERIPHERAL OEDEMA

Ascites (fluid building on your stomach hollow space, performing like a bulge throughout your tummy place) and peripheral oedema (swelling for your ankles and legs) are very not unusual in humans with superior cirrhosis. Ascites may be uncomfortable and make it tough for people to breathe and devour typically. In addition, there's a risk of infection in the fl uid, referred to as spontaneous bacterial peritonitis (SBP), which can be life threatening and is treated with antibiotics.

The primary treatments for ascites and oedema are sodium limit (low salt weight loss plan and diuretics, which include spironolactone and Furosemide). It may be helpful to peer a dietitian approximately a way to manage on this kind of strict diet. Some patients advantage from having the fluid drained off the stomach with a needle and tube. This usually needs to be repeated each few weeks. Patients considered at higher risk of contamination may be supplied prophylactic (preventative) antibiotics to take each day.

CHAPTER FIVE

HEPATIC ENCEPHALOPATHY

Many people with cirrhosis enjoy episodes of hepatic encephalopathy, most at a stage in which it isn't always very noticeable. In overt levels (wherein it's miles substantive), it can show up as sleep disturbance, mild confusion, diffused character modifications and slightly poorer performances in tests along with drawing a celebrity and connecting dots. It can also feature issues in movement (referred to as ataxia) and speech, slurring of phrases, tremor and a particular symptom of fl apping palms whilst you increase your hands (called asterixis). In a few humans the sleepiness can development to a lack of recognition and even to a coma, wherein it may be life-threatening.

The most important treatment for encephalopathy is lactulose (a candy syrupy medicine). This no longer only acts as a laxative however additionally enables the frame dispose of the pollutants that increase within the frame while the liver is failing. People are given sufficient lactulose so that they have one or loose bowel moves each day. They will also be given different laxatives and/ or an enema. Most durations of encephalopathy are brought on by problems along with an contamination, constipation, dehydration, a remedy or a bleed. It is essential that sufferers are seeking scientific advice so the reason of an episode can be diagnosed and dealt with.

BLEEDING

The liver makes merchandise to help blood clot (inclusive of clotting factors and platelets) and when the liver stops operating successfully, sufferers may be at risk of severe bleeding. Treatments encompass administering nutrition K and plasma in scientific emergencies. People have to are looking for expert advice before having clinical methods, which include any dental paintings, and make sure that they deal with any cuts that bleed with stress and bandages and seek medical help.

KIDNEY TROUBLES

People with decompensated cirrhosis who're already very sick with problems inclusive of encephalopathy, jaundice and bleeding troubles, are susceptible to a serious worry called hepatorenal syndrome, that's kidney failure in liver disease. For maximum patients, a liver transplant is needed, for a few urgently.

LIVER CANCER

Some people with cirrhosis develop liver cancer, most typically hepatocellular carcinoma (HCC). The intention is to come across and treat liver most cancers as early as possible.

Treatment can involve slicing out the a part of the liver stricken by most cancers. There are a ramification of different remedies aimed toward controlling the most cancers, such as injections of chemotherapy, radio frequency ablation and oral drugs. A liver transplant may be an option for a few sufferers.

LIVER TRANSPLANTATION

If your liver may be very badly broken, a liver transplant may be needed. This is a method in which a diseased liver is eliminated all through a lengthy operation and changed with a wholesome donor liver.

A liver transplant is usually only endorsed if different treatments are now not beneficial and your lifestyles is threatened through cease stage liver sickness. It is a major operation and you'll want to plan it cautiously together with your medical crew, own family and buddies.

Liver transplantation is generally very successful despite the fact that in a few cases it's far feasible for liver sicknesses to go back and have an effect on your new liver.

Discuss any issues you've got approximately your suitability for remedy together with your expert nurse or doctor and people nearest to you.

Looking after yourself Day-to-day coping techniques

In widespread, it's miles great to goal for as close to a regular lifestyles as viable. However, there are a few points that you need to hold in mind to help you feel as wholesome as you can.

• Take care of yourself by ensuring sufficient relaxation and workout.

• Follow practical hygiene measures if your immunity is low.

• Always discuss the use of over-the-counter tablets along with your medical doctor considering the fact that it's far vital to keep away from a few, in particular painkillers inclusive of aspirin and ibuprofen, when you have cirrhosis.

• Try to restrict your exposure to colds and other infectious illnesses.

• Talk in your physician about having a flu vaccination within the wintry weather months.

• Before travelling abroad, speak on your health practitioner about whether you have to have any vaccinations.

• Join a support group for greater information and personal support.

• Take an active hobby on your healthcare.

• Gather as a whole lot information as you want from charity phone help lines and their assisting websites.

If you discover yourself turning into depressed, communicate this over with your doctor who can talk ways of overcoming this. If appropriate, sure medicinal drugs may be useful in supporting you cope. Remember that liver characteristic can enhance in case you take care of yourself and receive early remedy. However, you must ensure that health professionals know you have cirrhosis earlier than giving or prescribing any treatment or medicine for you.

CHAPTER SIX

DIET

It is critical to eat nicely and to consist of a very good balance of foods to your weight-reduction plan consisting of nutrients, minerals and calcium. It is probable you will want extra electricity and protein.

Cirrhosis influences your capability to keep glycogen, a carbohydrate that offers you quick-term power. This approach that your frame has to apply its own muscle tissues to offer energy between meals and this may result in muscle wasting and weak point.

If you are affected on this way, snacking among meals is a manner you could top up on calories and protein. Another accurate approach is to consume 3 or 4 small food in an afternoon instead of one huge protein or carbohydrate-heavy meal.

You may additionally locate having nourishing beverages a help. These can include homemade milkshakes or commercially-made merchandise such as Build Up, Complan, Recovery and Nourishment. These are available at most chemists. It is a superb idea to test with your health practitioner or dietician first to make sure they are appropriate for you.

Try to avoid salty ingredients or including salt to what you consume, to assist control fluid retention.

ALCOHOL AND CIRRHOSIS

Almost everyone who liquids an excessive amount of alcohol will go through some liver damage, however this does not always turn into cirrhosis. As many as 9 out of ten folks who drink to excess will broaden a fatty liver, with one in ten progressing to cirrhosis.

In general, the greater you drink, the greater your danger of growing alcohol associated hepatitis or cirrhosis. A bad weight-reduction plan may make the hassle worse.

All forms of alcoholic liquids can cause liver disorder. If you have cirrhosis – whether it's miles resulting from alcohol or not – you ought to no longer drink alcohol in any respect.

TREATMENTS FOR LIVER DAMAGE

Abstinence is tried first. Several pills, including a few antioxidants (which include S-adenosyl-L-methionine, phosphatidylcholine, and metadoxine) and capsules to reduce infection, can be beneficial, however further examine is needed. Many dietary dietary supplements which can be antioxidants, which includes milk thistle and nutrients A and E, had been attempted but are useless.

Corticosteroids can assist relieve severe liver inflammation and are secure to apply if people do no longer have an infection, bleeding inside the digestive tract, kidney failure, or pancreatitis.

Liver transplantation may be finished if the damage is severe. Transplantation enables human beings to stay longer. However, due to the fact about half of the humans begin ingesting again after transplantation, most transplantation packages require that human beings be abstinent for six months to qualify.

ABSTINENCE

Abstinence is commonly the first-rate remedy. Other than liver transplantation, abstinence is the simplest treatment that could sluggish or reverse alcoholic liver ailment. In addition, it's miles available to all and has no aspect effects.

Because abstinence is hard, numerous techniques are used to assist inspire humans and to assist them change their behaviour. Strategies consist of behavioural therapy and psychotherapy (speak remedy)—regularly as part of a formal rehabilitation program—in addition to self-help and guide groups (including Alcoholics Anonymous) and counselling periods with the primary care medical doctor. Therapies that explore and help human beings clarify why they want to abstain from alcohol (referred to as motivational enhancement remedy) may also be used.

CHAPTER SEVEN

DRUGS

Drugs are once in a while used however most effective to complement behavioral and psychosocial healing procedures (see Detoxification and rehabilitation). Some capsules (consisting of naltrexone, nalmefene, baclofen, or acamprosate) assist by means of lowering withdrawal symptoms and the longing for alcohol. Disulfiram allows because it reasons unpleasant signs and symptoms (consisting of flushing) while humans take it and then drink alcohol. However, disulfiram has not been shown to promote abstinence and therefore is usually recommended most effective for positive people.

TREATMENT OF SYMPTOMS AND HEADACHES

Doctors deal with the troubles caused by alcoholic liver disease and the withdrawal symptoms that increase after humans stop consuming.

A nutritious diet and nutrition dietary supplements (in particular B nutrients) are vital at some stage in the first few days of abstinence. They can assist accurate dietary deficiencies that may cause headaches including weak point, shaking, loss of sensation and energy, anemia, and Wernicke encephalopathy. Supplements can also improve widespread fitness. Often, if irritation is severe, humans are hospitalized and can need to be fed through a tube to acquire ok nutrition.

Benzodiazepines (sedatives) are used to treat withdrawal symptoms (see

Emergency remedy). However, if alcoholic liver ailment is advanced, sedatives are used in small doses or prevented due to the fact they can cause port systemic encephalopathy.

PROGNOSIS

The analysis depends on how a whole lot fibrosis and inflammation are gift.

If humans prevent drinking and no fibrosis is gift, fatty liver and inflammation can be reversed. Fatty liver may additionally completely clear up inside 6 weeks. Fibrosis and cirrhosis often cannot be reversed.

Certain biopsy and blood take a look at results can assist doctors predict a person's analysis better. Doctors can also use formulas and models (which combine diverse take a look at outcomes) to help are expecting prognosis.

Once cirrhosis and its headaches (along with fluid accumulation inside the stomach and bleeding within the digestive tract) expand, the diagnosis is worse. Only about half of the humans with those headaches are nonetheless alive after 5 years. People who prevent consuming generally tend to live longer than people who do now not stop consuming.

Treatment

•	Stopping ingesting (abstinence) and assistance in doing so

•	Treatment of signs and headaches

•	Treatments for liver harm.

THE END